The Vegan Bodybuilders Diet

The ultimate 40 quick and easy recipes to improve your health with low carbon high protein foods, grow muscle, increase energy and live a healthy life.

Daniel Wilson

Test of Contents

Introduction

The plant-based diet is one of the most efficient ways to lose weight. It is better than another non-vegetarian dieting with vegans giving the best results. It takes a lot of self-discipline and patience to follow the diet, but in the end, all that is rewarded with your goals being achieved.

You need to plan if you are thinking about dieting. First, you can start slowly by just eating one meal a day, which is vegetarian and gradually increasing your number of vegetarian meals. Whenever you are struggling, ask your friend or family member to support you and keep you motivated. One important thing is also to be regularly accountable for not following the diet.

If dieting seems very important to you and you need to do it right, then it is recommended that you visit a professional such as a nutritionist or dietitian to discuss your dieting plan and optimizing it for the better.

No matter how much you want to lose weight, it is not advised that you decrease your calorie intake to an unhealthy level. Losing weight does not mean that you stop eating. It is done by carefully planning meals.

A plant-based diet is very easy once you get into it. At first, you will start to face a lot of difficulties, but if you start slowly, then you can face all the barriers and achieve your goal.

Healthy plant-derived protein tends to be high in vitamins, minerals, fiber, antioxidants and various other substances that we require to remain healthy and balanced. Some kinds include considerable quantities of healthy and balanced fats, as well. Beans, nuts, seeds and entire groups of grains are all healthy plant proteins that you should consume.

Research studies have revealed that healthy plant protein, as part of a plant-based diet plan, lowered the body weight and enhanced insulin resistance in obese individuals. If you are looking to reach your healthy and balanced weight, including even more plants to your diet plan is a terrific step, to begin with.

The next step is to decide how and when you are going to make the switch. Whether you choose to do it slowly, or you prefer to jump right in, the important thing is that you have made the decision. Within a short time, you should notice many positive changes and improvements in how your body feels and responds during periods of physical activity. You should see how much better you are able to train and compete as well as feel much better overall.

At first, it may take a little bit of getting used to, once you have switched to the fully vegan diet. Though, it will not take long for your body to eliminate all of the "bad stuff". Once this happens, you should notice that you have made the right decision, not only for your health, but also to improve your sports performance.

Start making changes in your diet. It's in your hands now. You have the facts about veganism and bodybuilding, and now it is up to you to decide how you are going to make the switch. It's a big switch to make, too, but it is completely doable. I like to suggest that you start with eating vegan two to three times a week and eat the way you are used to the rest of the week, for a month or so. This can help you get familiarize to your new diet and will help your body to adjust.

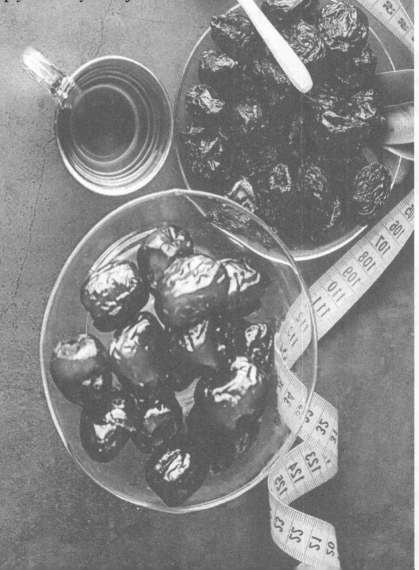

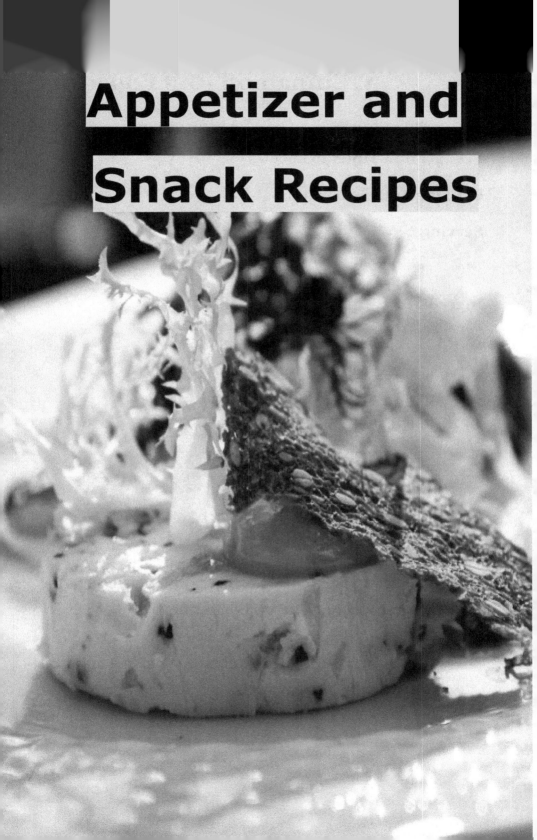

Appetizer and
Snack Recipes

1. Cinnamon Roll Popcorn

Preparation Time: 10 minutes

Cooking Time: 0 minutes

Servings: 3

Ingredients:

- 2 teaspoons vegetable oil
- 1/3 cup popcorn kernels
- 2 tablespoons coconut palm sugar
- ½ teaspoon ground cinnamon
- 2 tablespoons vegan butter
- 1 tablespoon maple syrup

Directions:

1. Use the vegetable oil in a large pan with a lid to make the popcorn according to package instructions.
2. Once the popcorn is popped, place the coconut palm sugar, cinnamon, butter and maple syrup in a saucepan over medium high heat. Stir constantly until everything melts and is well combined.

3. Place the popcorn in a large bowl and drizzle the sauce over the top. Toss with two large spoons to combine and let it cool before serving.

Nutrition:

195 Calories

3.8g Fiber

2.5g Protein

2.Pumpkin Flavored Popcorn

Preparation Time: 5 minutes

Cooking Time: 10 minutes

Servings: 10

Ingredients:

- 10 cups popped popcorn
- 2 tablespoons maple syrup
- 2 tablespoons coconut oil, melted
- 1 tablespoon pumpkin puree
- ¼ teaspoon cinnamon
- ½ teaspoon salt

Direction:

1. Make the popcorn and place it in a large bowl, reserving two cups of the popcorn to be placed in a four-cup measuring cup.
2. Preheat the oven to 325 degrees, Fahrenheit.

3. In a small saucepan, combine the maple syrup, coconut oil, puree, cinnamon and salt and put over medium heat. Stir constantly while it cooks, for about two minutes.

4. Put all the popcorn except the reserved two cups into a large roasting pan lined with aluminum foil.

5. Drizzle sauce over the popcorn in the roasting pan and stir until it is all coated.

6. Place in the oven for eight minutes, stirring every two or three minutes.

7. Remove from oven and let it cool; the popcorn will harden.

8. Pour the two cups of plain popcorn on top and stir to break up the hardened popcorn and incorporate all together.

Nutrition:

66 Calories

1.2g Fiber

1.1g Protein

3. Quinoa Tacos

Preparation Time: 10 minutes

Cooking Time: 1 hour

Serving: 6

Ingredients:

- 1 cup quinoa
- ¾ cup water
- 1 cup vegetable broth
- 1 tablespoon nutritional yeast
- ½ cup salsa
- ½ teaspoon garlic powder
- 2 teaspoons chili powder
- 2 teaspoon cumin
- ½ teaspoon sea salt
- ½ teaspoon ground pepper
- 1 tablespoon olive oil

Direction:

1. Rinse the quinoa and drain.
2. Preheat saucepan over medium heat and toast the quinoa for about four minutes stirring constantly.
3. Boil water and vegetable broth.
4. Simmer, cover and cook for 17 minutes. Fluff with a fork, put the lid back on and set to cool 10 minutes.
5. Prepare the oven to 375 degrees Fahrenheit and cover a shallow sided baking sheet with aluminum foil.
6. Place the cooled quinoa in a mixing bowl and add the nutritional yeast, salsa, garlic powder, chili powder, cumin, salt, pepper and oil and stir to combine.
7. Spread on prepared baking sheet and bake 20 minutes, stir around in the pan and bake another 20 minutes.
8. Serve in taco shells or on tostadas.

Nutrition:

149 Calories

3.2g Fiber

6.2g Protein

4.Vegan Caramel Popcorn

Preparation Time: 5 minutes

Cooking Time: 1 hour

Serves: 8

Ingredients:

- 8 cups popped popcorn
- ½ cup vegan butter
- 2/3 cups brown sugar
- 2 tablespoons agave nectar
- ¼ teaspoon baking soda
- 1 pinch salt
- 1 teaspoon vanilla

Direction:

1. Prep the oven to 250 degrees, Fahrenheit and line a baking sheet with parchment paper.
2. Spread the popped popcorn on the baking sheet and set it aside.
3. Over medium heat, cook the butter in pan.

4. Add the brown sugar and whisk constantly until it starts to bubble.
5. Add the agave nectar, baking soda, salt and vanilla and stir.
6. Once the foaming stops, pour it onto the popcorn and use a spatula to turn the popcorn while drizzling in a stream. Make sure all the corn is coated and pat smooth.
7. Bake for one hour, stirring it up every 15 minutes.

Nutrition:

180 Calories

1.2g Fiber

1.2g Protein

5. Zucchini Nuggets

Preparation Time: 5 minutes

Cooking Time: 40 minutes

Servings: 8

Ingredients:

- 7 small potatoes
- 2 medium zucchinis, grate
- ½ teaspoon sweet paprika
- ¼ teaspoon salt
- ¼ teaspoon ground pepper

Direction:

1. Cook the potatoes in boiling water. Drain and let them cool so they can be handled.
2. Ready the oven to 425 degrees, Fahrenheit and line two baking sheets with parchment paper. It is hard to get them all on one baking sheet, but the second may only be half full.

3. Grid the zucchini and squeeze out the liquid by wrapping it in a clean kitchen towel and twisting and squeezing. Place in a medium bowl.

4. Grate the cooked potatoes and place them in the bowl with the zucchini.

5. Add the paprika, salt and pepper, adjusting to your taste and mix with your hands.

6. Scoop out 1½ to two tablespoons of the mixture at a time and shape them into nuggets or tot shapes. Brush each one with olive oil on all sides. Place on baking sheets.

7. Bake for 35 to 40 minutes.

Nutrition:

111 Calories

3.7g Fiber

2.8g Protein

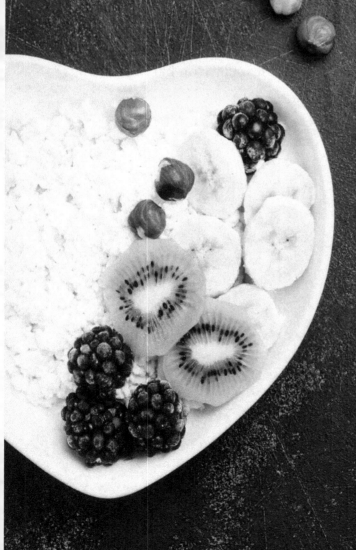

Breakfast

Recipes

6. Chickpeas on Toast

Preparation Time: 5 minutes

Cooking Time: 15 minutes

Servings: 6

Ingredients:

- 14-oz cooked chickpeas
- 1 cup baby spinach
- 1/2 cup chopped white onion
- 1 cup crushed tomatoes
- ½ teaspoon minced garlic
- ¼ teaspoon ground black pepper
- 1/2 teaspoon brown sugar
- 1 teaspoon smoked paprika powder
- 1/3 teaspoon sea salt
- 1 tablespoon olive oil
- 6 slices of gluten-free bread

Directions:

1. Situate frying pan, over medium heat, cook onion for 2 minutes.
2. Cook in garlic, for 30 seconds, stir in paprika and continue cooking for 10 seconds.
3. Stir in tomatoes, simmer the mixture, season with black pepper, sugar, and salt then add in chickpeas.
4. Add in spinach, cook for 2 minutes, then remove the pan from heat.
5. Serve cooked chickpeas on toasted bread.

Nutrition:

305 Calories

7.6g Fat

13g Protein

7. Peanut Butter Granola

Preparation Time: 10 Minutes

Cooking Time: 47 minutes

Servings: 4

Ingredients:

- 4 cups oats
- 1/3 cup of cocoa powder
- ¾ cup peanut butter
- 1/3 cup maple syrup
- 1/3 cup avocado oil
- 1½ teaspoons vanilla extract
- ½ cup cocoa nibs
- 6 ounces dark chocolate

Directions

1. Preheat your oven to 300 degrees F.
2. Spray a baking sheet with cooking spray.
3. In a medium saucepan add oil, maple syrup, and peanut butter.
4. Cook for 2 minutes on medium heat, stirring.

5. Add the oats and cocoa powder, mix well.

6. Spread the coated oats on the baking sheet.

7. Bake for 45 minutes, occasionally stirring.

8. Garnish with dark chocolate, cocoa nibs, and peanut butter.

Nutrition:

134 Calories

4.7g Fat

6.2g Protein

8.   Apple Chia Pudding

Preparation Time: 10 minutes

Cooking Time: 5 minutes

Servings: 4

Ingredients:

Chia Pudding:

- 4 tablespoons chia seeds
- 1 cup almond milk
- ½ teaspoon cinnamon

Apple Filling:

- 1 large apple
- ¼ cup water
- 2 teaspoons maple syrup
- Pinch cinnamon
- 2 tablespoons golden raisins

Directions

1. In a sealable container, add cinnamon, chia seeds and almond milk, mix well.
2. Seal the container and refrigerate overnight.
3. In a medium pot, combine all apple pie filling ingredients and cook for 5 minutes.
4. Serve the chia pudding with apple filling on top.

Nutrition:

387 Calories

2.9g Fiber

6.6g Protein

9.Pumpkin Spice Bites

Preparation Time: 10 minutes

Cooking Time: 0 minutes

Servings: 2

Ingredients:

- ½ cup pumpkin puree
- ½ cup almond butter
- ¼ cup maple syrup
- 1 teaspoon pumpkin pie spice
- 1 1/3cup rolled oats
- 1/3 cup pumpkin seeds
- 1/3 cup raisins
- 2 tablespoons chia seeds

Directions

1. In a sealable container, add everything and mix well.
2. Seal the container and refrigerate overnight.
3. Roll the mixture into small balls.
4. Serve.

Nutrition:

212 Calories

4.4g Fibers

7.3g Protein

10. Oatmeal with Black Beans & Cheddar

Preparation Time: 10 minutes

Cooking Time: 0 minute

Servings: 2

Ingredients:

- ½ cup rolled oats
- ¼ cup Greek yogurt
- ½ cup almond milk
- 2 tablespoons seasoned black beans
- 2 tablespoons Cheddar cheese
- 1 stalk scallion
- 1 tablespoon cilantro

Directions

1. Incorporate all the ingredients except the cilantro in a glass jar with lid.
2. Refrigerate for up to 5 days.
3. Sprinkle the cilantro on top before serving.

Nutrition:

47 Calories

1.2g fat

2g Protein

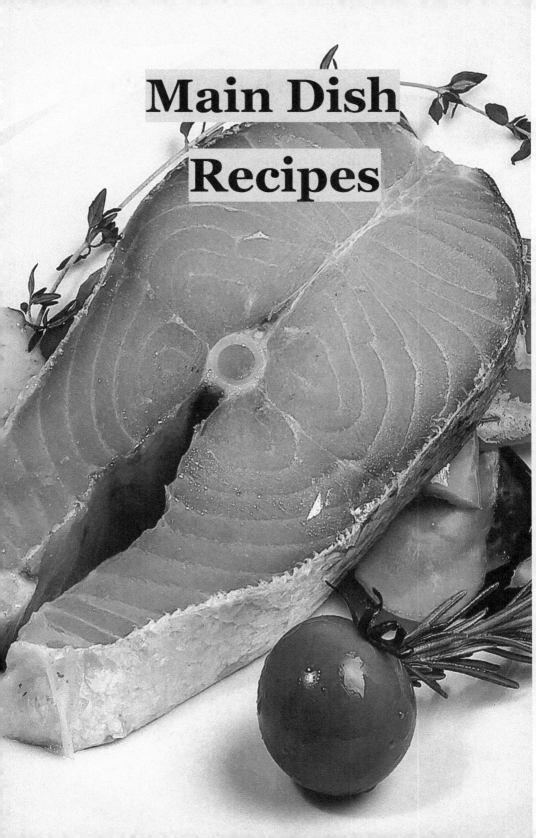

Main Dish

Recipes

11. Teriyaki Tofu Wraps

Preparation Time: 15 minutes

Cooking Time: 15 minutes

Serving: 3

Ingredients:

- 1 14-oz. package extra firm tofu
- 1 small white onion
- ½ pineapple
- ¼ cup soy sauce
- 2 tbsp. sesame oil
- 1 garlic clove
- 1 tbsp. coconut sugar
- 3-6 large lettuce leaves
- 1 tbsp. roasted sesame seeds

Direction:

1.   Take a medium-sized bowl and mix the soy sauce, sesame oil, coconut sugar, and garlic.

2.   Cut the tofu into ½-inch cubes, place them in the bowl, and marinate, up to 3 hours.

3. Meanwhile, cut the pineapple into rings or cubes.

4. After the tofu is adequately marinated, place a large skillet over medium heat, and pour in the tofu with the remaining marinade, pineapple cubes, and diced onions; stir.

5. Add salt and pepper to taste, making sure to stir the ingredients frequently, and cook until the onions are soft and translucent—about 15 minutes.

6. Divide the mixture between the lettuce leaves and top with a sprinkle of roasted sesame seeds.

7. Serve right away, or, store the mixture and lettuce leaves separately.

Nutrition

259 Calories

15g Fat

12g Protein

12. Tex-Mex Tofu & Beans

Preparation Time: 10 minutes

Cooking Time: 15 minutes

Serving: 4

Ingredients:

- 1 cup dry black beans
- 1 cup dry brown rice
- 1 14-oz. package firm tofu
- 2 tbsp. olive oil
- 1 small purple onion
- 1 medium avocado
- 1 garlic clove
- 1 tbsp. lime juice
- 2 tsp. cumin
- 2 tsp. paprika
- 1 tsp. chili powder

Direction:

1. Cook black beans following package directions.

2. Prepare the brown rice according to the recipe.

3. Cut the tofu into ½-inch cubes.

4. Cook olive oil and onion over high heat for 5 minutes.

5. Add the tofu and cook an additional 2 minutes, flipping the cubes frequently.

6. Meanwhile, cut the avocado into thin slices and set aside.

7. Set heat to medium and mix in the garlic, cumin, and cooked black beans.

8. Stir until everything is incorporated thoroughly, and then cook for 5 minutes.

9. Add the remaining spices and lime juice to the mixture in the skillet.

10. Mix thoroughly and remove the skillet from the heat.

11. Serve the Tex-Mex tofu and beans with a scoop of rice and garnish with the fresh avocado.

Nutrition

315 Calories

17g Fat

13g Protein

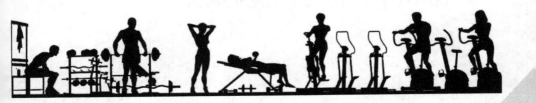

13. Vegan Friendly Fajitas

Preparation Time: 10 minutes

Cooking Time: 20 minutes

Serving: 6

Ingredients:

- 1 cup dry black beans
- 1 large green bell pepper
- 1 poblano pepper
- 1 large avocado
- 1 medium sweet onion
- 3 large Portobello mushrooms
- 2 tbsp. olive oil
- 6 tortilla wraps
- 1 tsp. lime juice
- 1 tsp. chili powder
- 1 tsp. garlic powder
- ¼ tsp. cayenne pepper
- Salt to taste

Direction:

1. Prep black beans.

2. Warm up olive oil in a frying pan over high heat.

3. Add the bell peppers, poblano peppers, and half of the onions.

4. Stir the chili powder, garlic powder, and cayenne pepper; add salt to taste.

5. Cook the vegetables until tender and browned, around 10 minutes.

6. Add the black beans and continue cooking for an additional 2 minutes; then remove the frying pan from the stove.

7. Add the portobello mushrooms to the skillet and turn heat down to low. Sprinkle the mushrooms with salt.

8. Stir/flip the ingredients often, and cook until the mushrooms have shrunk down to half their size, around 7 minutes. Remove the frying pan from the heat.

9. Mix the avocado, remaining 1 tablespoon of olive oil, and the remaining onions together in a small bowl to make a simple guacamole. Stir lime juice and season.

10. Top it with guacamole and scoop of the mushroom mixture.

Nutrition

264 Calories

14g Fat

6.8g Protein

14. Tofu Cacciatore

Preparation Time: 10 minutes

Cooking Time: 30 minutes

Serving: 3

Ingredients:

- 1 14-oz. package extra firm tofu
- 1 tbsp. olive oil
- 1 cup matchstick carrots
- 1 medium sweet onion
- 1 medium green bell pepper
- 1 28-oz. can dice tomatoes
- 1 4-oz. can tomato paste
- ½ tbsp. balsamic vinegar
- 1 tbsp. soy sauce
- 1 tbsp. maple syrup
- 1 tbsp. garlic powder
- 1 tbsp. Italian seasoning

Direction:

1. Chop the tofu into ¼- to ½-inch cubes.

2. Cook oil over medium-high heat.

3. Add the onions, garlic, bell peppers, and carrots; sauté for 10 minutes.

4. Now add the balsamic vinegar, soy sauce, maple syrup, garlic powder and Italian seasoning.

5. Stir well while pouring in the diced tomatoes and tomato paste; mix until all ingredients are thoroughly combined.

6. Add the cubed tofu and stir one more time.

7. Cover the pot, turn the heat to medium-low, and allow the mixture to simmer for 20-25 minutes.

Nutrition

274 Calories

10g Fat

14g Protein

15. Portobello Burritos

Preparation Time: 20 minutes

Cooking Time: 30 minutes

Serving: 4

Ingredients:

- 3 large Portobello mushrooms
- 2 medium potatoes
- 4 tortilla wraps
- 1 medium avocado
- ¾ cup salsa
- 1 tbsp. cilantro
- ½ tsp. salt

Marinade:

- 1/3 cup water
- 1 tbsp. lime juice
- 1 tbsp. minced garlic
- ¼ cup teriyaki sauce

Direction:

1. Prep oven to 400°F / 200°C.

2. Slightly grease a sheet pan with olive oil and set it aside.

3. Combine the water, lime juice, teriyaki, and garlic in a small bowl.

4. Slice the portobello mushrooms into thin slices and marinate thoroughly, for three hours.

5. Cut the potatoes. Sprinkle the fries with salt and then transfer them to the sheet pan. Place the fries in the oven and bake for 30 minutes. Flip once halfway through for even cooking.

6. Over medium heat, add the marinated mushroom slices with the remaining marinade to the pan. Cook until the liquid has absorbed, around 10 minutes. Remove from heat.

7. Fill the tortillas with a heaping scoop of the mushrooms and a handful of the potato sticks. Top with salsa, sliced avocados, and cilantro before serving.

8. Serve right away and enjoy, or, store the tortillas, avocado, and mushrooms separately for later!

Nutrition

239 Calories

9.2g Fat

5.1g Protein

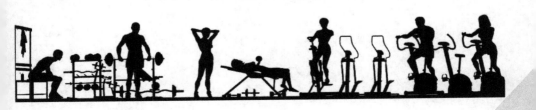

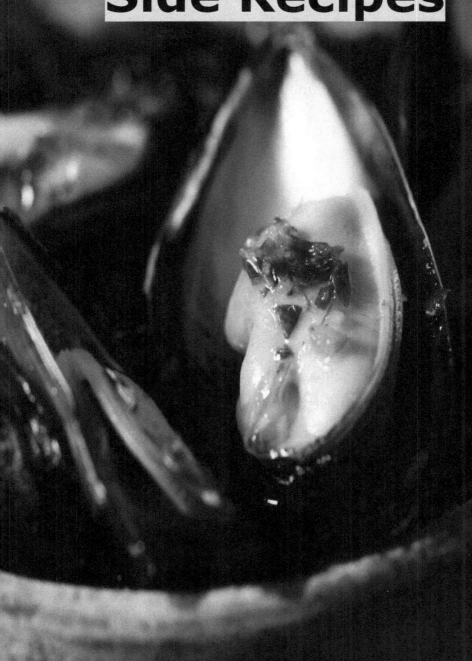

Side Recipes

16. Luscious Eggplant

Preparation Time: 5 minutes

Cooking Time: 16 minutes

Serving: 4

Ingredient:

- 1-pound eggplant
- 2½ cups water
- 20 small fresh curry leaves
- 4 teaspoons maple syrup
- 1 tablespoon tamari
- 3 large garlic cloves
- 2 teaspoons toasted sesame oil
- ¼ to ½ teaspoon red pepper flakes

Direction

1. Mix eggplant, water, and curry leaves (if using) over medium-high heat. Cook for 10 to 12 minutes, stirring occasionally, until the eggplant is tender. If the pan becomes dry before the eggplant is tender, add more water.

2. Add the maple syrup, tamari, garlic, oil, and red pepper flakes. Stir-fry for another 3 to 4 minutes. Serve immediately.

Nutrition:

44 Calories

2g Fat

1g Protein

17. Pizza Hummus

Preparation Time: 10 minutes

Cooking Time: 0 minute

Serving: 3

Ingredient

- 1 (15-ounce) can chickpeas
- 1 cup tomato sauce
- ¼ cup nutritional yeast
- ¼ cup water
- 3 tablespoons extra-virgin olive oil
- 3 large garlic cloves, peeled
- 1 tablespoon dried oregano
- 1 tablespoon dried rosemary
- 1 tablespoon dried basil
- 1 tablespoon balsamic vinegar
- 1 teaspoon sea salt

Direction

1. In a blender, combine the chickpeas, tomato sauce, nutritional yeast, water, oil, garlic, oregano, rosemary, basil, vinegar, and salt. Blend until completely smooth.
2. Garnished with basil and olives.

Nutrition:

223 Calories

8g Fat

6g Protein

18. Butter Bean Smash

Preparation Time: 5 minutes

Cooking Time: 3 minutes

Serving: 4

Ingredient

- 2 (15-ounce) cans butter beans
- 2 tablespoons plain unsweetened nondairy milk
- 4 teaspoons olive oil
- 4 teaspoons red wine vinegar
- 2 to 3 large garlic cloves
- ¾ teaspoon sea salt
- ¼ teaspoon freshly ground black pepper

Direction

1. In a medium pot, combine the beans, milk, oil, vinegar, garlic, salt, and pepper. Stir very well, until as "smashed" as possible
2. Heat over low heat for 3 minutes. Serve topped with the chives (if using).

Nutrition:

210 Calories

5g Fat

10g Protein

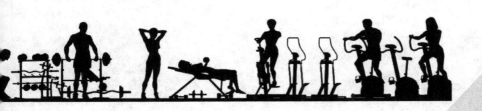

19. Chili-Ginger Cabbage

Preparation Time: 10 minutes

Cooking Time: 5 minutes

Serving: 5

- **Ingredient:**
- 6 cups finely chopped green cabbage
- ¼ cup water
- ¼ cup lime juice
- ¼ cup fresh ginger
- 3 tablespoons agave nectar
- 1 teaspoon red pepper flakes
- ¾ teaspoon sea salt

Direction

1. In a wok, sauté the cabbage in the water over medium-high heat, stirring often, for 5 minutes, or just until it becomes slightly wilted. Transfer to a large bowl.
2. Add the lime juice, ginger, agave, red pepper flakes, and salt to the bowl and stir well.

3. Chill for an hour or more. Stir well and serve cold or at room temperature

Nutrition:

63 Calories

1g Fat

2g Protein

20. Yellow Split Pea Rolls with Berbere Sauce

Preparation Time: 10 minutes

Cooking Time: 20 minutes

Serving: 8

Ingredient:

For rolls

- 16 spring roll rice paper wraps
- Ethiopian-Spiced Yellow Split Peas
- Nonstick cooking spray

For Berber Sauce

- 2 tablespoons neutral-flavored oil
- 2½ cups chopped white or yellow onions
- ¼ cup plus 2 tablespoons water
- 2 tablespoons berbere
- 1 teaspoon sea saltDirection

For rolls

1. Preheat the oven to 400°F.

2. Gently take a rice paper wrap and run it under warm water until thoroughly moistened on both sides. Lay flat on a nonporous surface and fill with about ¼ cup of the Ethiopian-Spiced Yellow Split Peas.

3. Wrap the bottom up and over the filling, then fold in the sides. Finish by rolling all the way up from the bottom, as if you were rolling a burrito. Repeat this process.

4. Situate rolls on a lightly oiled or nonstick baking sheet. Lightly spray the top of the rolls with cooking spray and bake for 15 to 20 minutes.

5. Let it cool, then serve with the berbere sauce for dipping.

For Berber sauce

1. While the rolls are cooking, in a large pan, heat the oil over medium heat and caramelize the onions in the oil for 10 to 20 minutes, stirring often. Remove from the heat and transfer to a blender.

2. Add the water, berbere, and salt and blend until very smooth.

Nutrition

177 Calories

5g Fat

3g Protein

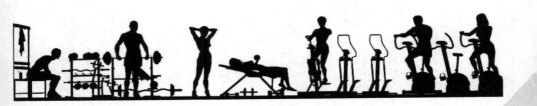

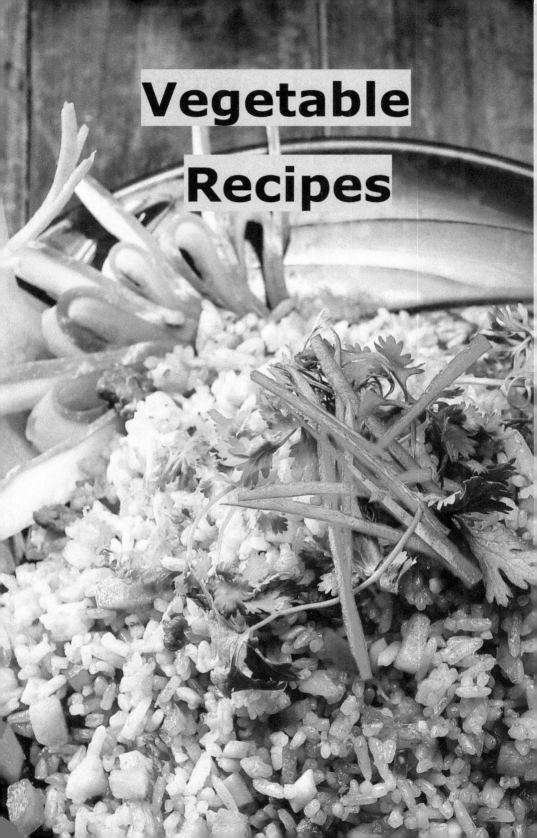

Vegetable

Recipes

21. Green Beans

Preparation Time: 15 minutes

Cooking Time: 20 minutes

Servings: 8

Ingredients:

- 1 shallot, chopped
- 24 oz. green beans
- Salt and pepper to taste
- ½ teaspoon smoked paprika
- 1 teaspoon lemon juice
- 2 teaspoons vinegar

Direction

1. Preheat your oven to 450 degrees F.
2. Stir in the shallot and beans.
3. Season with salt, pepper and paprika.
4. Roast for 10 minutes.
5. Drizzle with the lemon juice and vinegar.
6. Roast for another 2 minutes.

Nutrition:

49 Calories

3g Fiber

2.9g Protein

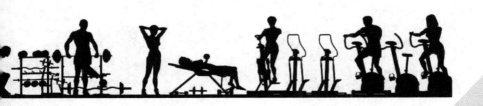

22. Coconut Brussels Sprouts

Preparation Time: 15 minutes

Cooking Time: 10 minutes

Servings: 4

Ingredients:

- 1 lb. Brussels sprouts, trimmed and sliced in half
- 2 tablespoons coconut oil
- ¼ cup coconut water
- 1 tablespoon soy sauce

Direction

1. In skillet over medium heat, stir the coconut oil and cook the Brussels sprouts for 4 minutes.
2. Pour in the coconut water.
3. Cook for 3 minutes.
4. Add the soy sauce and cook for another 1 minute.

Nutrition:

114 Calories

4.3g Fiber

4g Protein

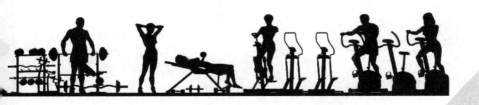

23. Creamy Polenta

Preparation Time: 5 minutes

Cooking Time: 45 minutes

Servings: 8

Ingredients:

- 1 1/3 cup cornmeal
- 6 cups water
- Salt to taste

Direction

1. Incorporate all the ingredients in a pan over medium high heat.
2. Boil and then simmer for 5 minutes.
3. Reduce the heat to low.
4. Stir until creamy for 45 minutes.
5. Let sit before serving.

Nutrition:

74 Calories: 74

3g Fiber

1.6g Protein

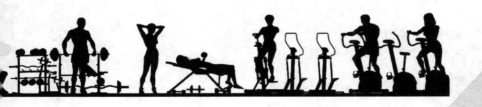

24. Skillet Quinoa

Preparation Time: 20 minutes

Cooking Time: 25 minutes

Servings: 4

Ingredients:

- 1 cup sweet potato, cubed
- ½ cup water
- 1 tablespoon olive oil
- 1 onion, chopped
- 3 cloves garlic, minced
- 1 teaspoon ground cumin
- 1 teaspoon ground coriander
- ½ teaspoon chili powder
- ½ teaspoon dried oregano
- 15 oz. black beans, rinsed and drained
- 15 oz. roasted tomatoes
- 1 ¼ cups vegetable broth
- 1 cup frozen corn
- 1 cup quinoa (uncooked)
- Salt to taste

- ½ cup light sour cream
- ½ cup fresh cilantro leaves

Direction

1. Add the water and sweet potato in a pan over medium heat.
2. Bring to a boil.
3. Decrease heat and cook sweet potatoes.
4. Add the oil and onion.
5. Cook for 3 minutes.
6. Cook garlic and spices for 1 minute.
7. Incorporate rest of the ingredients except the sour cream and cilantro.
8. Cook for 20 minutes.
9. Serve with sour cream and top with the cilantro before serving.

Nutrition:

421 Calories

11g Fiber

16g Protein

25. Green Beans with Balsamic Sauce

Preparation Time: 10 minutes

Cooking Time: 15 minutes

Servings: 6

Ingredients:

- 2 shallots, sliced
- 8 cups green beans, trimmed
- 2 tablespoons olive oil
- Salt and pepper to taste
- 2 tablespoons balsamic vinegar
- ¼ cup Parmesan cheese, grated

Direction

1. Preheat your oven to 425 degrees F.
2. Line your baking with foil.
3. In the pan, toss the shallots and beans in oil, salt and pepper.
4. Roast in the oven for 15 minutes.
5. Drizzle with the vinegar and top with cheese.

Nutrition:

78 Calories

0.6g Fiber

1.9g Protein

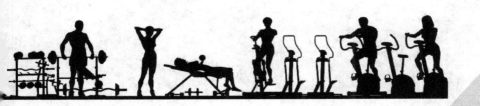

Soup and Stew Recipes

26. Broccoli Creamy Soup

Preparation Time: 5 minutes

Cooking Time: 15 minutes

Serving: 2

Ingredients:

- 3 cup Vegetable Broth
- 2 Green Chili
- 2 cups Broccoli Florets
- 1 tbsp. Chia Seeds
- 1 cup Spinach
- 1 tsp. Oil
- 4 Celery Stalk
- 1 Potato, medium & cubed
- 4 Garlic cloves
- Salt, as needed
- Juice of ½ of 1 Lemon

Direction:

1. First, heat the oil in a large sauté pan over a medium-high heat.
2. Once the oil becomes hot, add the potatoes to it.
3. When the potatoes become soft, stir all the remaining ingredients into the pan, excluding the spinach, chia seeds, and lemon.
4. Cook and then add the spinach and chia seed to the pan.
5. Put off the heat after cooking for 2 minutes.
6. Allow the spinach mixture to cool slightly. Fill mixture into a high-speed and blend for two minutes or until smooth.
7. Pour the lemon juice over the soup. Stir and serve immediately.
8. Enjoy.

Nutrition:

977 Calories

36g Protein

84g Carbohydrates

27. Chickpea and Sweet Potato Soup

Preparation Time: 10 minutes

Cooking Time: 25 minutes

Serving: 4

Ingredients:

- ½ tsp. Red Pepper Flakes
- 1 tsp. Extra Virgin Olive Oil
- 2 cups Vegetable Broth
- 2 Garlic cloves, minced
- ½ tsp. Cumin
- 1 White Onion, small & chopped
- 1 tbsp. Basil, fresh & chopped
- 1 Orange Bell Pepper, diced
- 1/8 tsp. Cinnamon
- 2 Carrots, large & diced
- 16 oz. can of Fire Roasted Diced Tomatoes
- 1 Sweet Potato, medium & diced
- 1 Avocado, sliced for garnish

Directions:

1. Start by heating a medium-sized pot over medium-high heat and to this spoon in the oil.
2. Once the oil becomes hot, stir in the onion, salt, and garlic. Mix well.
3. Cook them for 2 minutes and then add the carrot and pepper to it.
4. Sauté the onion mixture for another 5 minutes and then stir in the diced tomatoes.
5. Now, add all the remaining ingredients, excluding the sweet potato and basil to it.
6. Bring the veggie soup mixture to a boil and lower the heat.
7. Then, stir in the sweet potato to the mix and allow it to simmer for 8 to 10 minutes or until everything becomes tender.
8. Taste for seasoning and spoon in more salt and pepper as needed.
9. Garnish with basil and serve along with avocado slices.

Nutrition:

279 Calories

8g Proteins

36g Carbohydrates

28. Black Bean Nacho Soup

Preparation Time: 5 minutes

Cooking Time: 30 minutes

Serving: 4

Ingredients:

- 30 oz. Black Bean
- 1 tbsp. Olive Oil
- 2 cups Vegetable Stock
- ½ of 1 Onion, large & chopped
- 2 ½ cups Water
- 3 Garlic cloves, minced
- 14 oz. Mild Green Chilies, diced
- 1 tsp. Cumin
- 1 cup Salsa
- ½ tsp. Salt
- 16 oz. Tomato Paste
- ½ tsp. Black Pepper

Direction

1. For making this delicious fare, heat oil in a large pot over medium-high heat.
2. Once the oil becomes hot, stir in onion and garlic to it.
3. Sauté for 4 minutes or until the onion is softened.
4. Next, spoon in chili powder, salt, cumin, and pepper to the pot. Mix well.
5. Then, stir in tomato paste, salsa, water, green chilies, and vegetable stock to onion mixture. Combine.
6. Bing the mixture to a boil. Allow the veggies to simmer.
7. When the mixture starts simmering, add the beans.
8. Bring the veggie mixture to a simmer again and lower the heat to low.
9. Finally, cook for 15 to 20 minutes and check for seasoning. Add more salt and pepper if needed.
10. Garnish with the topping of your choice. Serve it hot.

Nutrition:

361 Calories

16g Proteins

53g Carbohydrates

29. Split Pea Vegetable Soup

Preparation Time: 10 minutes

Cooking Time: 60 minutes

Serving: 8

Ingredients:

- 1 Red Bell Pepper, chopped
- 2 tbsp. Olive Oil
- 8 cups Vegetable Broth
- 1 Sweet Onion, large & diced
- 3 White Potatoes, small & cubed
- Salt & Pepper, to taste
- 4 Garlic cloves, minced
- 2 cups Split Peas, dried
- 2 Bay Leaves
- 3 Carrot, sliced
- 1 tbsp. Parsley, dried
- 1 Pepper, chopped
- 1 tsp. Smoked Paprika
- 3 Celery Ribs, chopped

- 1 Red Bell Pepper, chopped

Direction:

1. For making this delightful soup, pour olive oil to a Dutch oven and heat it over medium-high heat.
2. Once the oil becomes hot, stir in onion, celery, pepper, garlic, and carrot to it.
3. Sweat the veggies for 5 minutes while stirring it frequently.
4. Then, spoon in all the spices to the pan. Mix.
5. Sauté the mixture for two minutes and then add split peas, broth, and potatoes to it.
6. Now, lower the heat and bring the mixture to a boil.
7. Cook for 1 hour while stirring it occasionally.
8. Pull out bay leaves and allow it to cool slightly.
9. Finally, blend the soup with a high-speed blender or with an immersion blender until you have smooth yet chunky soup.
10. Situate the soup back to the pot and taste for seasoning.
11. Warm the soup and serve it hot. Garnish with parsley.

Nutrition:

198 Calories

8g Proteins

5g Fat

30. Peanut Soup with Veggies

Preparation Time: 10 minutes

Cooking Time: 25 minutes

Serving: 3

Ingredients:

- 2 tbsp. Soy Sauce
- 1 cup Brown Rice
- 1 Garlic clove, minced
- ½ of 1 Red Onion, chopped
- 4 tbsp. Peanut Butter
- 1 Carrot, small & chopped
- 3 tbsp. Tomato Paste
- ½ of 1 Courgette, medium & chopped
- 3 cups Vegetable Broth
- ½ tbsp. Ginger, grated
- 2 tbsp. Peanuts
- Dash of Hot Sauce

Direction:

1. To begin with, boil the broth in a large saucepan over medium heat. Allow it to boil.
2. In the meantime, cook the rice by following the instructions given in the packet.
3. After that, stir in the onion, carrot, and courgette to the saucepan. Mix well.
4. Next, spoon in the ginger and garlic to the mixture.
5. Then, add the peanuts, tomato paste, and peanut butter to the pan. Combine.
6. Season and add soy sauce to it.
7. Now, allow it to simmer until the rice gets cooked.

Nutrition:

488 Calories

15g Proteins: 15g

15g Fat

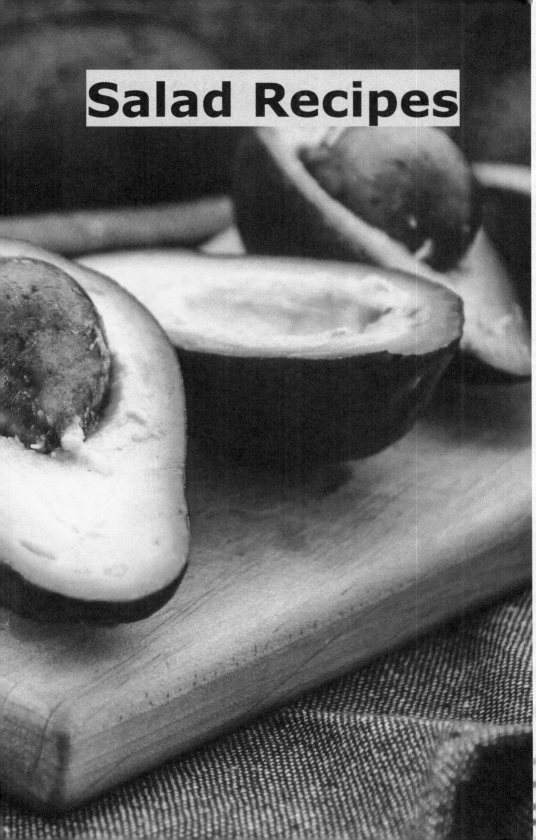

Salad Recipes

31. Pasta with Asparagus

Preparation Time: 15 minutes

Cooking Time: 12 minutes

Servings: 4

Ingredients

- ¼ cup olive oil
- 5 garlic cloves, minced
- ½ teaspoon red pepper flakes, crushed
- 1/8 teaspoon hot pepper sauce
- 1-pound asparagus
- Salt and ground black pepper, to taste
- ½ pound cooked whole-wheat pasta, drained

Direction

1.   In a large cast-iron skillet, heat the oil over medium heat and cook the garlic, red pepper flakes, and hot pepper sauce for about 1 minute.

2.   Add the asparagus, salt, and black pepper and cook for about 8–10 minutes, stirring occasionally.

3.   Place the hot pasta and toss to coat well.

4.   Serve immediately.

Nutrition

326 Calories

9g Fiber

12g Protein

32. Buddha Bowl

Preparation Time: 20 minutes

Cooking Time: 0 minute

Servings: 6

Ingredients

Dressing

- ¼ cup balsamic vinegar
- ¼ cup low-sodium soy sauce
- 2 tablespoons water
- 1 teaspoon sesame oil, toasted
- 1 teaspoon Sriracha
- 3–4 drops liquid stevia

Salad

- 3 cups canned chickpeas, rinsed and drained
- 1½ pounds baked firm tofu, cubed
- 2 large zucchinis, sliced thinly
- 2 large yellow bell peppers, seeded and sliced thinly

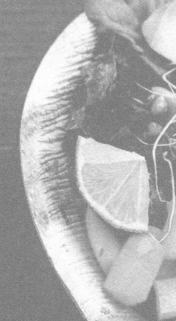

- 3 cups cherry tomatoes, halved
- 2 cups radishes, sliced thinly
- 2 cups purple cabbage, shredded
- 6 cups fresh baby spinach
- 2 tablespoons white sesame seeds

Direction

1. For dressing: in a bowl, add all the ingredients and beat until well combined.

2. Divide the chickpeas, tofu, and vegetables into serving bowls.

3. Drizzle with dressing and serve immediately with the garnishing of sesame seeds.

Nutrition

305 Calories

11g Fiber

21g Protein

33. Vegetarian Taco Bowl

Preparation Time: 15 minutes

Cooking Time: 0 minute

Servings: 2

Ingredients

- 2 teaspoons olive oil
- 1 red bell pepper, seeded and chopped
- 1 red onion, sliced
- 1 cup canned black beans, rinsed and drained
- ½ cup frozen corn, thawed
- 3 cups lettuce, chopped
- 1 jalapeño pepper, seeded and minced
- 1 tablespoon fresh lime juice
- ¼ cup salsa

Direction

1.   Divide the beans, corn, veggies, lettuce, and jalapeño pepper into serving bowls.

2.   Drizzle with lime juice and serve alongside the salsa.

Nutrition

257 Calories

10g Fiber

11g Protein

34. Chickpeas with Swiss Chard

Preparation Time: 15 minutes

Cooking Time: 15 minutes

Servings: 4

Ingredients

- 2 tablespoons olive oil
- 1 medium yellow onion, chopped
- 4 garlic cloves, minced
- 1 teaspoon dried thyme, crushed
- 1 teaspoon dried oregano, crushed
- ½ teaspoon paprika
- 1 cup tomato, chopped finely
- 2½ cups canned chickpeas, rinsed and drained
- 5 cups Swiss chard
- 2 tablespoons water
- 2 tablespoons fresh lemon juice
- Salt and ground black pepper, to taste
- 3 tablespoons fresh basil, chopped

Direction

1.   Heat the olive oil in a skillet over medium heat and sauté onion for about 6–8 minutes.

2.   Add the garlic, herbs, and paprika and sauté for about 1 minute.

3.   Add the Swiss chard and 2 tablespoons water and cook for about 2–3 minutes.

4.   Add the tomatoes and chickpeas and cook for about 2–3 minutes.

5.   Add in the lemon juice, salt, and black pepper, and remove from the heat.

6.   Serve hot with the garnishing of basil.

Nutrition

260 Calories

9g Fiber

12g Protein

35. Chickpeas with Veggies

Preparation Time: 15 minutes

Cooking Time: 35 minutes

Servings: 6

Ingredients

- 2 (15-ounce) cans chickpeas
- 5 sweet potatoes, peeled and cubed
- 2 tablespoons olive oil
- 1 teaspoon dried basil, crushed
- ½ teaspoon garlic powder
- Salt and ground black pepper, to taste
- 3 cups fresh baby spinach

Direction

1.   Preheat the oven to 425°F. Line a baking dish with parchment paper.

2.   In a large bowl, add all ingredients (except for spinach) and toss to coat well. Spread chickpea mixture onto the prepared baking dish in a single layer.

3.   Bake for about 30–35 minutes, stirring after every 10 minutes.

4.   Remove from the oven and immediately, stir in the spinach.

5.   Cover the baking dish for about 5 minutes before serving.

Nutrition

344 Calories

11g Fiber

11g Protein

Dessert Recipes

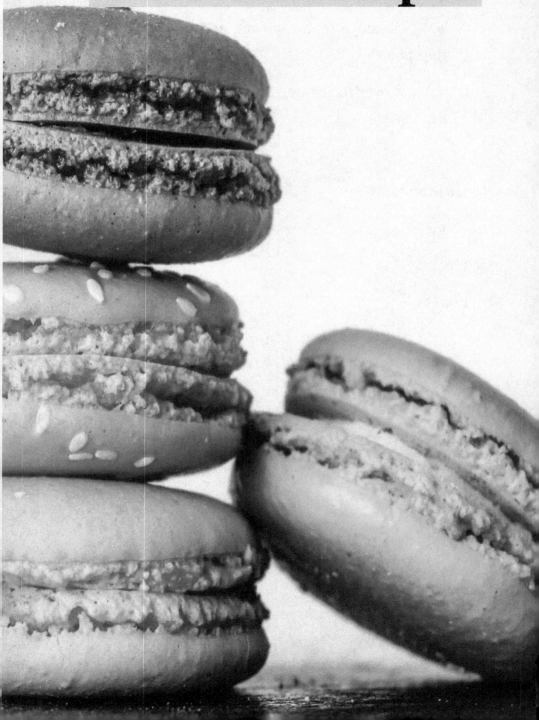

36. Zucchini Chocolate Crisis Bread

Preparation Time: 15 minutes

Cooking Time: 25 minutes

Serving: 8

Ingredients:

- 1 cup sugar
- 2 tbsp. flax seeds
- 6 tbsp. water
- 1 cup applesauce
- 1/3 cup cocoa powder
- 2 cups all-purpose flour
- 2 tsp. vanilla
- 1 tsp. baking soda
- ½ tsp. baking powder
- 1 tbsp. cinnamon
- 1 tsp. salt
- 2 1/3 cup grated zucchini
- 1 cup nondairy chocolate chips

Directions:

1. Begin by preheating your oven to 325 degrees Fahrenheit.
2. First, mix together the water and the flax seeds and allow the mixture to thicken to the side for five minutes.
3. Mix all the dry ingredients together. Next, add the wet ingredients to the dry ingredients, including the flax seeds. Next, add the chocolate chips and the zucchini. Stir well, and spread the batter out into your bread loaf pan. Bake the creation for thirty minutes. Afterward it cools, enjoy!

Nutrition

116 Calories

4g Fat

8g Protein

37. Banana Blueberry Bread

Preparation Time: 15 minutes

Cooking Time: 35 minutes

Servings: 8

Ingredients:

- 3 tbsp. lemon juice
- 4 bananas
- ½ cup agave nectar
- ½ cup vegan milk
- 1 ¾ cup all-purpose flour
- 1 tsp. baking soda
- 1 tsp. baking powder
- 1 tsp. salt
- 2 cups blueberries

Directions:

1. Begin by preheating your oven to 350 degrees Fahrenheit.
2. Next, mix together the dry ingredients in a large bowl and your wet ingredients in a different, smaller bowl. Make sure to mash up the bananas well.
3. Stir the ingredients together in the large bowl, making sure to assimilate the ingredients together completely. Add the blueberries last, and then pour the mixture into a bread pan. Allow the bread to bake for fifty minutes, and enjoy.

Nutrition

119 Calories

7g Fat

11g Protein

38. Vegan Apple Cobbler Pie

Preparation Time: 15 minutes

Cooking Time: 25 minutes

Serving: 3

Ingredients:

- 3 cups sliced apples
- 6 cups sliced peaches
- 2 tbsp. arrowroot powder
- ½ cup white sugar
- 1 tsp. cinnamon
- 1 tsp. vanilla
- ½ cup water

Biscuit Topping Ingredients:

- ½ cup almond flour
- 1 cup gluten-free ground-up oats
- ½ tsp. salt
- 2 tsp. baking powder

- 2 tbsp. white sugar
- 1 tsp. cinnamon
- ½ cup soymilk
- 4 tbsp. vegan butter

Directions:

1. Begin by preheating your oven to 400 degrees Fahrenheit.
2. Next, coat the peaches and the apples with the sugar, arrowroot, the cinnamon, the vanilla, and the water in a large bowl. Allow the mixture to boil in a saucepan. After it begins to boil, allow the apples and peaches to simmer for three minutes. Remove the fruit from the heat and add the vanilla.
3. You've created your base.
4. Now, add the dry ingredients together in a small bowl. Cut the biscuit with the vegan butter to create a crumble. Add the almond milk, and cover the fruit with this batter.
5. Bake this mixture for thirty minutes. Serve warm, and enjoy!

Nutrition

116 Calories

7g Fat

16g Protein

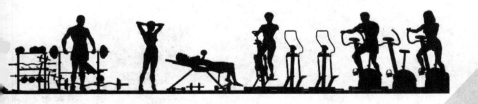

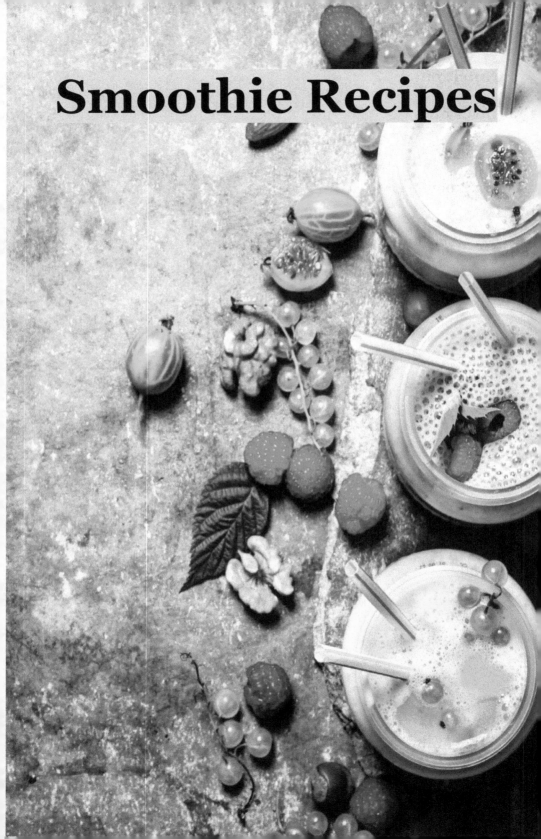

Smoothie Recipes

39. Nice Spiced Cherry Cider

Preparation Time: 5 minutes

Cooking Time: 4 hours

Servings: 16

Ingredients:

- 2 cinnamon sticks, each about 3 inches long
- 6-ounce of cherry gelatin
- 4 quarts of apple cider

Directions:

1. Using a 6-quarts slow cooker, pour the apple cider and add the cinnamon stick.
2. Stir, then cover the slow cooker with its lid. Plug in the cooker and let it cook for 3 hours at the high heat setting or until it is heated thoroughly.
3. Then add and stir the gelatin properly, then continue cooking for another hour.
4. When done, remove the cinnamon sticks and serve the drink hot or cold.

Nutrition:

100 Calories

2g Carbohydrates

5g Protein.

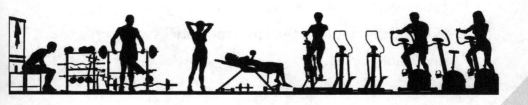

40. Fragrant Spiced Coffee

Preparation Time: 10 minutes

Cooking Time: 3 hours

Servings: 8

Ingredients:

- 4 cinnamon sticks, each about 3 inches long
- 1 1/2 teaspoons of whole cloves
- 1/3 cup of honey
- 2-ounce of chocolate syrup
- 1/2 teaspoon of anise extract
- 8 cups of brewed coffee

Directions:

1. Pour the coffee in a 4-quarts slow cooker and pour in the remaining ingredients except for cinnamon and stir properly.
2. Wrap the whole cloves in cheesecloth and tie its corners with strings.
3. Soak cheesecloth bag in the slow cooker and cover it with the lid.

4. Turn on slow cooker and cook on low heat setting for 3 hours.
5. When done, discard the cheesecloth bag and serve.

Nutrition:

150 Calories

35g Carbohydrates

3g Protein

Conclusion

Thanks for making it to the end of this guide.

A plant-based diet provides a simple, effective way to cut processed foods from your diet. As well as being in my mind, healthier than animal-based products, plant-based products are cheaper. Plus, as long as you eat the appropriate variety, it's likely that a plant-based diet is nutritionally sufficient. Moreover, a plant-based diet is more ethical than an animal-based diet. The grain fed to livestock could be feeding humans. Animals have to endure a lifetime on factory farms. Plants however don't endure anything. They grow and then die. They don't produce waste or pollution. They don't consume any resources. It should be pretty clear that a plant-based diet is, environmentally speaking, the way we should eat. Still, individuals often assume a plant-based diet isn't complete enough unless you add in the meat.

It's easy to assume that humans aren't likely to thrive without adding meat. But it turns out that we're doing just fine. For example, many of the wealthiest countries have diets that are heavily plant-based—yet they also have among the lowest rates of diet-related diseases. Unlike plants, animals are used for meat, milk, and eggs. But those products only provide a small fraction of the essential nutrients for optimal health. The majority of protein a healthy person need comes from plants.

Animal protein is no different in this regard. Simply by switching to a plant-based diet you will soon discover that you can still get enough protein—even if you're a meat-eater. However, plant protein is far superior to animal protein. The proteins in animal products increase the risk of breast cancer, prostate cancer, cardiovascular disease, diabetes, and other illnesses.

Plant protein, on the other hand, reduces the risks of those diseases. The protein in plants is high in fiber and low in saturated fat. A plant-based diet is also rich in antioxidants—particularly vitamin C. Plant-based antioxidants actually reduce cholesterol levels. They also help the body deal with heat stress and provide support for the immune system.

In a nutshell, a plant-based diet is far more fulfilling than animal-based products. Although a plant-based diet may seem more expensive than animal-based products, this isn't the case. The meat, dairy and egg industries are heavily subsidized with public money. This makes their products cheap. Meanwhile, plants are often priced according to how much water and fuel they require. As a result, many of the world's population pays more for animal products than they would for plants. A plant-based diet is healthier and more environmentally sound—as well as more ethical. What's not to love?

Humans have long enjoyed eating plant-based food. Even the earliest hunter-gatherers ate increasingly fewer plants as they started hunting more and more animals. Over time, plant-based food became rarer and rarer among the world's meat-eating communities. As a result, plant-based food is now considered a luxury in much of the world. People may not consider it luxurious, but animals certainly do. They don't actually care what they eat. They don't choose to be eaten any more than we choose to eat plants. They don't even know our language. But needless to say, we wouldn't employ, slaughter and eat animals like we currently do if we tried to think like them.

If we took an animal's perspective, the way we raise animals for food would be repulsive. Despite the fact that this is what animals think—and that the way we treat them is painful and unfair, we still believe we have the right to consume them and use them for material gain. If we were to look at the situation from an animal's perspective, the only conclusion to be drawn is that we have no right to exploit them for our own consumption—let alone the consumption of their own families. Although some individuals have now embraced a plant-based diet, the vast majority of people still consume an animal-based diet.

CPSIA information can be obtained
at www.ICGtesting.com
Printed in the USA
BVHW091030260421
605864BV00003B/555